Regina J. Butts

Healing in Time

Learning to Trust the Process of
Healing with Time

Regina J. Butts

Regina J. Butts

Regina J. Butts

Table Of Contents

Chapter 1: Introduction

- The importance of healing

- The role of time in healing

Chapter 2: Understanding the Healing Process

- The stages of healing

- Common obstacles to healing

Chapter 3: Why Time is a Key Component of Healing

- How time helps us process emotions and experiences

- The benefits of giving ourselves time to heal

Chapter 4: Embracing Patience and Trusting the Process

- Letting go of the need for instant results

- Cultivating trust in the natural process of healing

Chapter 5: Tools and Techniques for Supporting Healing with Time

- Self-care practices for emotional and physical healing

- Therapeutic interventions that support the healing process

Chapter 6: Common Challenges to Trusting the Process

- Coping with impatience and frustration

- Dealing with setbacks and relapses

Conclusion

- The power of healing with time

- Encouragement to trust the process and prioritize self-care

Chapter 1

Introduction

Healing is a fundamental aspect of our human experience. We all experience pain, whether physical or emotional, and we all seek relief from it. Yet, the process of healing is not always straightforward, and it can be easy to become frustrated or discouraged along the way. This is where the role of time in healing becomes so important.

Time is an essential component of the healing process. It allows us to process our emotions and experiences, to gain perspective and insight, and to learn new coping mechanisms. However, in our fast-paced and instant gratification-focused society, it can be challenging to give ourselves the time we need to truly heal. We may feel pressure to "get over it" quickly, or we may compare our healing journey to others and feel inadequate if we're not progressing as quickly as we think we should.

We'll explore the concept of healing with time and learn how to trust the natural process of healing. We'll delve into the stages of healing, discuss common obstacles that can impede progress, and look at why time is so crucial to the healing process. We'll also explore some practical tools and techniques for supporting our healing journey and address common challenges that can arise when trying to trust the process.

Ultimately, the goal of this article is to encourage and empower readers to prioritize their healing and embrace patience and trust as they navigate the ups and downs of the healing process. By the end, readers should have a better understanding of how time can support their healing journey and a range of practical strategies for making the most of this essential component of the healing process.

As we dive deeper into the concept of healing with time, it's important to acknowledge that healing is not a linear process. It's not something that can be neatly compartmentalized or measured with a stopwatch. Rather, healing is messy, nonlinear, and deeply personal. Each person's journey is unique, and there is no "right" or "wrong" way to heal.

However, there are certain patterns and stages that tend to emerge in the healing process. These may include denial, anger, bargaining, depression, and acceptance, or they may take on different forms depending on the individual and the specific circumstances of their healing journey. By understanding these stages, we can better prepare ourselves for what lies ahead and be more compassionate and understanding towards ourselves as we navigate them.

One of the reasons why time is so important in the healing process is that it allows us to move through these stages at our own pace. We can't rush or force ourselves to feel better. Healing requires patience, self-compassion, and a willingness to sit with discomfort and uncertainty.

At the same time, there are practical steps we can take to support our healing with time. These may include self-care practices such as exercise, healthy eating, meditation, and journaling, as well as therapy, support groups, or other therapeutic interventions. It's important to remember that these practices are not a cure-all, and they may not work for everyone. However, they can provide helpful tools and strategies for managing difficult emotions and processing experiences in a healthy and constructive way.

Of course, trusting the process of healing with time is not always easy. We may feel frustrated, stuck, or overwhelmed at times, and we may experience setbacks or relapses along the way. It's important to acknowledge these challenges and give ourselves permission to feel what we feel. We can't always control the external factors that impact our healing journey, but we can control how we respond to them.

Healing with time is not just about "getting over it" or "moving on." It's about acknowledging our pain, honoring our experiences, and taking the time we need to heal in a way that feels authentic and meaningful to us. It's about trusting that we have the inner resources and resilience to navigate difficult times and emerge stronger and more whole on the other side.

The importance of healing

Healing is an essential aspect of our human experience. It allows us to recover from physical and emotional pain, to restore our sense of well-being and balance, and to regain our strength and vitality.

Physical healing is perhaps the most obvious form of healing. When we suffer an injury or illness, our body naturally goes into a process of healing. Our immune system kicks into gear, repairing damaged tissue and fighting off infection.

Over time, our body gradually returns to a state of health and balance, and we're able to resume our normal activities.

Emotional healing, on the other hand, can be more elusive and complex. It often requires us to confront and process difficult emotions, such as grief, anger, or shame, and to work through past traumas or painful experiences. Emotional healing may take longer than physical healing, and it may require ongoing support and self-care. However, the rewards of emotional healing can be profound. When we're able to heal from emotional pain, we may experience greater self-awareness, resilience, and a deeper sense of connection with others.

The importance of healing extends beyond our individual well-being. When we're able to heal from our own pain, we're better able to show up for others with empathy, compassion, and understanding. We're able to create healthier relationships and communities, and to be a positive force for change in the world.

Unfortunately, the importance of healing is often overlooked or undervalued in our culture. We may feel pressure to push through our pain, to "tough it out," or to ignore our emotions altogether. We may view healing as a sign of weakness or as a luxury that we can't afford. However, in reality, healing is an essential aspect of our overall health and well-being, and it's something that deserves our attention and care.

By prioritizing our healing, we're able to honor our experiences, process our emotions in a healthy way, and ultimately emerge stronger and more resilient. Whether we're healing from physical or emotional pain, the process of healing is not always easy, but it's ultimately a worthwhile and transformative journey.

Healing is essential to our physical, emotional, and spiritual well-being. It involves a process of recovering from an injury, illness, or trauma, and restoring balance to our body, mind, and spirit. The importance of healing cannot be overstated, as it allows us to regain our strength, vitality, and resilience.

Six reasons why healing is important

1. Promotes Physical Health: Healing is important for promoting physical health. When we experience injuries or illnesses, our body's natural healing process kicks in to restore the injured tissues and fight off infections.

Proper rest, nutrition, and medical care can support this process and help us recover fully.

2. Enhances Emotional Well-being: Healing is also important for enhancing our emotional well-being. Trauma, loss, and other life challenges can leave emotional wounds that require healing. By addressing these wounds and working through our emotions, we can find greater peace, joy, and fulfillment in life.

3. Builds Resilience: Healing builds resilience, which is the ability to bounce back from adversity. By overcoming challenges and healing from past injuries or trauma, we become stronger and more resilient. This resilience can help us navigate future challenges

with greater ease and confidence.

4. Improves Relationships: Healing can also improve our relationships with others. When we heal from past wounds, we can let go of resentment, anger, and other negative emotions that may be impacting our relationships. We can also communicate more effectively and build deeper connections with others.

5. Supports Personal Growth: Healing supports personal growth by providing an opportunity for self-reflection and self-improvement. By addressing our past wounds and working through our emotions, we can gain a greater understanding of ourselves and our values. This self-awareness can help us make

positive changes in our lives and pursue our goals with greater clarity and purpose.

6. Enhances Spiritual Connection: Healing can enhance our spiritual connection by bringing us closer to our true selves and our higher power. By addressing past wounds and working through our emotions, we can find greater peace, meaning, and purpose in life. This can lead to a deeper sense of spiritual connection and fulfillment.

Healing is essential to our well-being and can bring many benefits to our physical, emotional, and spiritual health. By recognizing the importance of healing and taking steps to promote our own healing, we can lead more fulfilling and satisfying lives.

The role of time in healing

The role of time in healing is critical. While some physical injuries may heal in a relatively short time, many emotional and psychological wounds require more extended periods for complete healing. Time enables the body to rest and recover, the mind to process emotions, and the spirit to gain new perspectives.

The major five roles of time in healing are:

1. Processing Emotions: After experiencing trauma or emotional pain, time allows us to process our emotions fully. It provides an opportunity to reflect on what happened, understand our feelings, and find ways to cope with them.

2. Physical Healing: Many physical

injuries require time to heal. Rest and recovery time can promote healing and prevent further injury.

3. Self-Reflection: Time provides space for self-reflection. By examining our thoughts, feelings, and behaviors, we can gain new insights into ourselves, our relationships, and our goals.

4. Building Resilience: Healing often requires resilience, which is built over time by practicing coping skills, adapting to new situations, and developing a long-term perspective.

5. Closure: Time can bring closure to a difficult experience. By taking time to process our emotions, reflect on our experiences, and find ways to move forward, we can

find peace and closure, which can be essential for our emotional and psychological well-being.

By recognizing the critical role of time in the healing process and allowing ourselves to take the time we need to heal fully, we can lead more fulfilling and satisfying lives.

Chapter 2

Understanding the Healing Process

Understanding the healing process is essential for anyone who wants to heal from emotional or physical trauma. Healing is a complex process that involves physical, emotional, and psychological components, and it can take time. Here are some key points to keep in mind when trying to understand the healing process:

1. Healing is a Process: Healing is not an event that happens suddenly. It is a process that involves multiple stages, and each stage requires a different approach. Accepting that healing takes time is essential to avoid becoming discouraged

during the process.

2. Healing is Unique to Each Person: Every person's healing process is unique. People experience different traumas and have different backgrounds, personalities, and experiences. Therefore, what works for one person may not work for another. It is essential to find an approach that is tailored to the individual.

3. Healing Requires Patience: Healing is not something that can be rushed. It takes time to process emotions, recover physically, and gain new perspectives. Rushing the process may lead to relapse or further injury.

4. Healing Involves Setbacks: Setbacks are a natural part of the

healing process. It is common to experience moments of doubt or frustration during the healing process. However, setbacks should not discourage individuals from continuing to move forward with the process.

5. Healing is Holistic: Healing involves the body, mind, and spirit. To heal fully, all three components must be addressed. Taking care of one aspect of healing while neglecting others may lead to an incomplete healing process.

6. Healing is Possible: It is important to remember that healing is possible. With patience, perseverance, and the right support, anyone can heal from emotional or physical trauma. There is hope, and the process can

be transformative.

Understanding the healing process is essential for anyone who wants to heal from emotional or physical trauma. Healing is a complex process that involves multiple stages, and it takes time. However, with patience, perseverance, and the right support, anyone can heal and lead a fulfilling life.

Stages of healing

The healing process involves several stages, and understanding these stages can be helpful in navigating the process. While the specifics of the stages can vary depending on the type of injury or trauma, here are the general stages of healing:

1. Hemostasis: The first stage of healing involves stopping bleeding and the formation of a blood clot

at the site of the injury. This process prevents further blood loss and reduces the risk of infection.

2. Inflammatory: The second stage involves inflammation, which helps to clean the wound by removing any debris or foreign objects. Inflammation also signals the immune system to send white blood cells to the site of the injury to fight infection and promote healing.

3. Proliferative: The third stage is characterized by the growth of new tissue, blood vessels, and skin. This stage is crucial for the formation of healthy tissue and the restoration of function.

4. Remodeling: The final stage of

healing involves remodeling the new tissue to match the surrounding tissue's strength and flexibility. This stage can take several months or even years, depending on the extent of the injury.

While the physical healing process can take time, it is essential to note that the emotional healing process can also involve stages. Here are some common emotional healing stages:

1. Shock and Denial: The initial stage of emotional healing often involves shock and denial. Individuals may feel numb or disconnected from their emotions as a way to cope with the trauma.

2. Anger and Depression: As individuals begin to process their

emotions, they may experience feelings of anger or depression. These emotions can be overwhelming but are a natural part of the healing process.

3. Acceptance: Over time, individuals may come to accept what has happened and begin to find ways to move forward. This stage involves finding meaning and purpose in the experience and learning to live with any physical or emotional scars.

Understanding the stages of healing can be helpful in navigating the process. The physical healing process involves hemostasis, inflammatory, proliferative, and remodeling stages. Emotional healing can also involve stages such as shock and denial, anger and depression, and acceptance. With time, patience, and the right support, individuals can heal from emotional and physical trauma and find meaning and purpose in their experiences.

Common obstacles to healing

Healing from emotional or physical trauma is a complex and challenging process that can involve many obstacles. These obstacles can be external or internal and may prevent individuals from achieving complete healing. Here are some common obstacles to healing:

1. Fear: Fear is a common obstacle to healing. Fear of the unknown, fear of the future, and fear of reliving past traumas can prevent individuals from taking steps toward healing.

2. Shame and guilt: Feelings of shame and guilt can be barriers to

healing. Individuals may blame themselves for what happened, and this can prevent them from seeking help or taking steps toward healing.

3. Lack of support: Lack of support from friends, family, or healthcare providers can make the healing process more challenging. Support from others is essential for individuals to feel validated, understood, and encouraged throughout the healing process.

4. Self-doubt: Self-doubt can be a significant obstacle to healing. Individuals may question their ability to heal or feel like they do not deserve to heal.

5. Trauma triggers: Trauma triggers are events or situations that

remind individuals of their trauma. These triggers can make healing more challenging, and individuals may need to learn coping strategies to manage them.

6. Physical limitations: Physical limitations, such as chronic pain or limited mobility, can make the healing process more challenging. These limitations can make it harder for individuals to participate in activities that promote healing or engage in self-care practices.

Healing from emotional or physical trauma can involve many obstacles. Fear, shame, lack of support, self-doubt, trauma triggers, and physical limitations are some common barriers to healing. However, with the right support and coping strategies, individuals can

overcome these obstacles and achieve
complete healing.

Chapter 3

Why Time is a Key Component of Healing

Healing from emotional or physical trauma can be a complex and challenging process, and time is a key component in the healing journey. Time can allow for physical healing, emotional processing, and the integration of new coping strategies. Here are some reasons why time is a key component of healing:

1. Physical Healing: Time is necessary for the body to heal physically. It takes time for wounds to close, bones to mend, and scars to form. The healing process cannot be rushed, and the body needs time to restore itself to full health.

2. Emotional Processing: Emotional healing takes time, and individuals need space and time to process their emotions fully. Rushing the emotional healing process can lead to unresolved trauma, which can lead to additional stress and health problems.

3. Integration of Coping Strategies: Healing often involves learning new coping strategies to manage stress and anxiety. Time is necessary to integrate these new strategies into daily life fully. This can involve practicing new habits, learning new skills, and incorporating new perspectives into one's life.

4. Perspective: Time can also provide a new perspective on the healing process. It can allow individuals to

see how far they have come and provide a sense of hope and encouragement for the future.

5. Patience: Healing requires patience, and time can provide an opportunity for individuals to cultivate patience and self-compassion. Rushing the healing process can lead to additional stress and setbacks.

Time is a crucial component of the healing journey. Physical healing, emotional processing, integration of new coping strategies, gaining perspective, and cultivating patience are some of the reasons why time is a vital aspect of healing. It is important to be patient and give oneself the time necessary to fully heal from emotional and physical trauma.

How time helps us process emotions and experiences

Time is a crucial factor in helping us process emotions and experiences. When we experience traumatic events or emotions, it is essential to allow ourselves the time and space to process them fully. Here are some ways in which time helps us process emotions and experiences:

1. Emotional Distance: Time provides us with emotional distance from a traumatic event or emotion. It allows us to step back and view the situation more objectively, which can aid in the healing process.

2. Clarity: With time, we can gain clarity on our emotions and experiences. We can look back on

past events and recognize patterns or triggers that contributed to our emotions.

3. Perspective: As time passes, we can gain a new perspective on past experiences. We may see how far we have come or recognize that what seemed insurmountable at the time is now manageable.

4. Acceptance: Time can also help us come to terms with our emotions and experiences. We may learn to accept what has happened and find ways to move forward.

5. Coping: Time can provide an opportunity to develop new coping strategies. We may try different techniques or seek out help from professionals, friends, or family members.

6. Integration: Finally, time allows us to integrate our emotions and experiences into our lives. We can learn from them, grow, and use them to create a more fulfilling future.

Time plays a crucial role in our ability to process emotions and experiences. It provides us with emotional distance, clarity, perspective, acceptance, coping strategies, and integration. By giving ourselves the time and space necessary to process our emotions and experiences, we can achieve healing and growth.

The benefits of giving ourselves time to heal

Giving ourselves time to heal is essential for our mental and physical well-being. It can be tempting to rush the healing process and try to move on quickly, but taking the time we need to heal can have many benefits. Here are some of the benefits of giving ourselves time to heal:

1. Reduced Stress: Taking the time we need to heal can reduce stress and anxiety. Rushing the healing process can lead to additional stress and setbacks, which can make the healing journey more challenging.

2. Increased Self-Awareness: When we take the time to heal, we can increase our self-awareness. We can learn more about our emotions, triggers, and coping mechanisms, which can help us better manage stress and anxiety in the future.

3. Improved Relationships: Taking the time we need to heal can also

improve our relationships with others. When we take care of ourselves and prioritize our healing, we can be more present and engaged with our loved ones.

4. Enhanced Resilience: Giving ourselves time to heal can enhance our resilience. By taking the time we need to recover from difficult experiences, we can develop the skills and strategies necessary to manage future challenges.

5. Improved Physical Health: Taking the time we need to heal can also improve our physical health. Stress and anxiety can have a negative impact on our physical health, and taking the time to heal can help reduce these negative effects.

6. Increased Creativity: Finally, taking the time we need to heal can increase our creativity. When we are not consumed by stress and anxiety, we may have more mental space to be creative and explore new ideas.

Giving ourselves time to heal is essential for our well-being. It can reduce stress, increase self-awareness, improve relationships, enhance resilience, improve physical health, and increase creativity. By prioritizing our healing and giving ourselves the time we need to recover from difficult experiences, we can achieve greater mental and physical well-being.

Chapter 4

Embracing Patience and Trusting the Process

Embracing patience and trusting the process are essential components of the healing journey. Healing takes time, and it is not a linear process. It can be challenging to trust the process and have patience when we are in pain or facing difficult emotions. However, here are some reasons why embracing patience and trusting the process is important:

1. Healing Takes Time: As discussed earlier, healing takes time. It is not something that can be rushed, and trying to do so can hinder the healing process. Embracing patience and trusting the process

allows us to take the time we need to fully heal and recover.

2. Trusting Ourselves: Embracing patience and trusting the process also involves trusting ourselves. It means having confidence in our ability to heal and knowing that we have the strength and resilience to overcome difficult emotions and experiences.

3. Mindfulness: When we embrace patience and trust the process, we can be more present and mindful. We can focus on the present moment and be fully aware of our emotions and surroundings. This can help us better manage stress and anxiety.

4. Reduced Anxiety: When we trust the process and embrace patience,

we can reduce anxiety. We can let go of the need for control and surrender to the healing journey. This can help us feel more calm and at peace.

5. Personal Growth: Finally, embracing patience and trusting the process can lead to personal growth. The healing journey can be a transformative experience, and by embracing patience and trusting the process, we can learn more about ourselves, develop new coping mechanisms, and grow as individuals.

Embracing patience and trusting the process are crucial components of the healing journey. It allows us to take the time we need to heal, trust ourselves, be present, reduce anxiety, and experience personal growth. By embracing patience and trusting the process, we can achieve greater mental and physical well-being.

Letting go of the need for instant results

Letting go of the need for instant results is an important aspect of the healing journey. We live in a fast-paced society that values quick fixes and instant gratification, which can make it challenging to embrace the slower pace of the healing process. However, here are some reasons why letting go of the need for instant results is crucial:

1. Healing Takes Time: As we have discussed earlier, healing takes time. It is not something that can be rushed or forced. Letting go of

the need for instant results allows us to take the time we need to fully heal and recover.

2. Reduced Stress: Letting go of the need for instant results can also reduce stress. Trying to force healing or expecting instant results can create additional stress and anxiety. By letting go of this need, we can reduce stress and focus on the healing journey.

3. Improved Self-Awareness: Letting go of the need for instant results can also improve self-awareness. We can learn more about our emotions, triggers, and coping mechanisms by being present in the moment and embracing the healing process.

4. Trusting the Process: Letting go of

the need for instant results also involves trusting the process. It means having faith in the healing journey and knowing that we will eventually achieve the results we desire.

5. Personal Growth: Finally, letting go of the need for instant results can lead to personal growth. The healing journey can be a transformative experience, and by embracing the process and letting go of the need for instant results, we can learn more about ourselves and develop new coping mechanisms.

Letting go of the need for instant results is an important aspect of the healing journey. It allows us to take the time we need to heal, reduce stress, improve self-awareness, trust the process, and experience personal growth. By embracing the slower pace of the healing journey, we can achieve greater mental and physical well-being.

Cultivating trust in the natural process of healing

Cultivating trust in the natural process of healing is an essential aspect of the healing journey. It involves having faith in our body's ability to heal itself, both physically and emotionally. When we trust the natural process of healing, we can let go of the need for control and embrace the journey with patience and openness. Here are some ways to cultivate trust in the natural process of healing:

1. Accepting the Present Moment: Cultivating trust in the natural process of healing requires

accepting the present moment, including our current physical and emotional state. Acceptance allows us to let go of resistance and begin the healing process from a place of peace and openness.

2. Letting Go of Control: Trusting the natural process of healing also involves letting go of the need for control. We cannot force healing or control the outcome, but we can control our attitude and approach to the healing journey.

3. Focusing on Self-Care: Taking care of ourselves physically and emotionally is an essential part of the healing journey. By prioritizing self-care, we can support our body's natural healing process and develop a deeper connection with

ourselves.

4. Practicing Mindfulness: Practicing mindfulness, such as meditation or breathing exercises, can help us cultivate trust in the natural process of healing. Mindfulness allows us to stay present in the moment, observe our thoughts and emotions without judgment, and develop a deeper sense of awareness.

5. Seeking Support: Finally, seeking support from loved ones, professionals, or support groups can also help us cultivate trust in the natural process of healing. Having a supportive network can provide encouragement, guidance, and accountability throughout the healing journey.

Cultivating trust in the natural process of healing involves accepting the present moment, letting go of control, focusing on self-care, practicing mindfulness, and seeking support. By embracing the healing journey with patience and openness, we can develop a deeper connection with ourselves and trust in the natural process of healing.

Chapter 5

Tools and Techniques for Supporting Healing with Time

Healing with time can be a challenging journey, but there are many tools and techniques that can support the healing process. These tools and techniques can help us process our emotions, develop self-awareness, and cultivate resilience. Here are some of the tools and techniques for supporting healing with time:

1. Journaling: Writing down our thoughts and emotions can be a powerful tool for processing our experiences and gaining self-awareness. Journaling can also help us track our progress and identify patterns in our healing

journey.

2. Mindfulness Practices: Mindfulness practices, such as meditation, deep breathing, or yoga, can help us develop a deeper connection with ourselves and stay present in the moment. These practices can also help us manage stress and anxiety, which can be obstacles to healing.

3. Therapy: Seeking support from a therapist or counselor can provide a safe space for exploring our emotions and experiences. Therapy can also help us develop coping skills and strategies for managing difficult emotions.

4. Self-Care Practices: Practicing self-care, such as getting enough sleep, eating nutritious foods, and

engaging in physical activity, can support our physical and emotional health. Self-care practices can also help us develop a deeper sense of self-compassion and self-love.

5. Creative Expression: Engaging in creative activities, such as art or music, can provide a powerful outlet for expressing our emotions and experiences. Creative expression can also help us develop a sense of self-awareness and self-discovery.

6. Gratitude Practices: Practicing gratitude, such as writing down three things we are grateful for each day, can help us develop a more positive outlook on life. Gratitude practices can also help us shift our focus away from

negative experiences and emotions and towards the positive aspects of our lives.

There are many tools and techniques for supporting healing with time. These tools and techniques can help us process our emotions, develop self-awareness, and cultivate resilience. By incorporating these practices into our daily lives, we can support our healing journey and develop a deeper sense of self-compassion and self-love.

Self-care practices for emotional and physical healing

Self-care practices are essential for both emotional and physical healing. Taking care of ourselves can help us manage stress, regulate our emotions, and improve our overall well-being. Here are some self-care practices for emotional and physical healing:

1. Get enough sleep: Getting adequate sleep is essential for our physical and emotional health. Sleep helps our bodies repair and regenerate, and it also helps us manage stress and regulate our emotions.

2. Eat nutritious foods: Eating a balanced diet with plenty of fruits, vegetables, lean protein, and healthy fats can support our physical and emotional health. Nutritious foods can help us feel more energized and focused and can also boost our mood.

3. Engage in physical activity: Exercise is an excellent way to support both physical and emotional healing. Exercise can

help us manage stress, regulate our emotions, and improve our physical health.

4. Practice relaxation techniques: Relaxation techniques, such as deep breathing, meditation, or yoga, can help us manage stress and anxiety. These techniques can also help us regulate our emotions and develop a sense of inner peace and calm.

5. Spend time in nature: Spending time in nature can be a powerful tool for emotional and physical healing. Nature can help us feel more grounded and connected to ourselves and the world around us.

6. Connect with loved ones: Building strong connections with loved ones can provide a source of

support and comfort during difficult times. Spending time with friends and family can also help us regulate our emotions and boost our mood.

Self-care practices are essential for emotional and physical healing. By taking care of ourselves, we can manage stress, regulate our emotions, and improve our overall well-being. Incorporating self-care practices into our daily lives can support our healing journey and help us cultivate a deeper sense of self-compassion and self-love.

Therapeutic interventions that support the healing process

Therapeutic interventions are professional treatments that can support the healing process. These interventions can help individuals process trauma, manage symptoms of mental health disorders, and develop coping strategies for everyday stressors. Here are some therapeutic interventions that support the healing process:

1. Talk therapy: Talk therapy, also known as psychotherapy, is a type of therapy that involves talking with a trained mental health professional. Talk therapy can help individuals process their thoughts and emotions, develop coping strategies, and work through traumatic experiences.

2. Cognitive-behavioral therapy (CBT): CBT is a type of therapy that focuses on changing negative thought patterns and behaviors. CBT can be used to treat a variety

of mental health disorders, including anxiety and depression.

3. Eye movement desensitization and reprocessing (EMDR): EMDR is a type of therapy that is used to treat trauma and post-traumatic stress disorder (PTSD). EMDR involves recalling traumatic experiences while simultaneously engaging in eye movements or other forms of bilateral stimulation.

4. Mindfulness-based interventions: Mindfulness-based interventions, such as mindfulness-based stress reduction (MBSR), involve developing awareness of the present moment and accepting one's thoughts and emotions without judgment. Mindfulness-based interventions can help

individuals manage stress and regulate their emotions.

5. Art therapy: Art therapy involves using creative expression to process thoughts and emotions. Art therapy can be helpful for individuals who have difficulty verbalizing their emotions or experiences.

6. Body-based therapies: Body-based therapies, such as yoga or somatic experiencing, focus on the relationship between the mind and body. These therapies can help individuals develop awareness of their physical sensations and use the body as a tool for healing.

Therapeutic interventions can be a valuable tool for supporting the healing process. Talk therapy, CBT, EMDR, mindfulness-based interventions, art therapy, and body-based therapies are just a few examples of interventions that can help individuals process trauma, manage symptoms of mental health disorders, and develop coping strategies for everyday stressors. It is important to work with a trained professional to determine which therapeutic interventions are most appropriate for one's individual needs.

Chapter 6

Common Challenges to Trusting the Process

Trusting the healing process can be challenging for many reasons. Here are some common challenges to trusting the process:

1. Fear: Fear of the unknown or fear of reliving past trauma can make it difficult to trust the process of healing. It can be tempting to avoid confronting painful emotions, but avoiding them can prevent progress in the healing process.

2. Impatience: It's common to want to see immediate results when working through difficult emotions or experiences. However, healing

is a gradual process and it's important to give yourself time to work through it.

3. Doubt: Doubting the effectiveness of the healing process or one's ability to heal can be a major obstacle. It's important to remind oneself that healing is possible and that progress can be made with time and effort.

4. Lack of support: Having a support system can make a big difference in the healing process. If you don't have people in your life who can provide emotional support, consider seeking out a therapist or support group.

5. Negative self-talk: Negative self-talk can create a self-fulfilling prophecy and hinder progress in

the healing process. It's important to challenge negative thoughts and practice self-compassion.

6. Lack of self-care: Prioritizing self-care is essential for the healing process. Neglecting self-care can make it difficult to manage stress and emotions, which can interfere with the healing process.

Trusting the process of healing can be challenging, but it's important to confront these challenges in order to make progress. Fear, impatience, doubt, lack of support, negative self-talk, and lack of self-care are common challenges that can hinder progress in the healing process. By recognizing these challenges and actively working to overcome them, individuals can make meaningful progress in their healing journey.

Coping with impatience and frustration

Dealing with impatience and frustration while healing is a common challenge. Here are some coping strategies to help manage impatience and frustration:

1. Practice mindfulness: Mindfulness can help individuals stay present and focused on the moment, instead of worrying about the future or dwelling on the past. It can also help individuals become more aware of their emotions and thoughts, which can help them manage impatience and frustration.

2. Set realistic goals: Setting realistic goals can help individuals feel a sense of accomplishment and progress. However, it's important

to remember that healing is a gradual process and progress may not always be linear.

3. Celebrate small victories: Celebrating small accomplishments along the way can help individuals stay motivated and positive.

4. Practice self-compassion: It's important to be kind and understanding towards oneself during the healing process. Practicing self-compassion can help individuals manage impatience and frustration.

5. Take breaks: Taking breaks from the healing process can be beneficial. It's important to take time to recharge and do things that bring joy and relaxation.

6. Seek support: Seeking support from loved ones, a therapist, or a support group can help individuals manage impatience and frustration. It can also provide an opportunity to discuss challenges and receive encouragement and validation.

Coping with impatience and frustration is a common challenge during the healing process. Mindfulness, setting realistic goals, celebrating small victories, practicing self-compassion, taking breaks, and seeking support are strategies that can help manage impatience and frustration. By using these strategies, individuals can stay motivated and make progress towards their healing goals.

Dealing with setbacks and relapses

Dealing with setbacks and relapses is a common challenge during the healing process. Here are some coping strategies to help manage setbacks and relapses:

1. Accept that setbacks and relapses are a natural part of the healing process: Setbacks and relapses are a normal part of the healing process. It's important to accept that setbacks can happen and that they don't mean that the healing process has failed.

2. Identify triggers: Identifying triggers that can lead to setbacks and relapses can help individuals avoid them or prepare for them. For example, if stress is a trigger, individuals can practice stress-management techniques or create a plan for managing stressors.

3. Seek support: Seeking support from loved ones, a therapist, or a support group can help individuals manage setbacks and relapses. It can also provide an opportunity to discuss challenges and receive encouragement and validation.

4. Reframe setbacks and relapses as opportunities for growth: Setbacks and relapses can provide opportunities for growth and learning. By reframing setbacks as opportunities to learn and grow, individuals can gain a sense of control and motivation to continue the healing process.

5. Practice self-compassion: It's important to be kind and understanding towards oneself during setbacks and relapses. Practicing self-compassion can

help individuals manage negative thoughts and emotions and stay motivated to continue the healing process.

6. Adjust expectations: Adjusting expectations during setbacks and relapses can help individuals avoid feelings of failure or disappointment. It's important to remember that setbacks and relapses don't mean that progress isn't being made.

Dealing with setbacks and relapses is a common challenge during the healing process. Accepting setbacks as a natural part of the process, identifying triggers, seeking support, reframing setbacks as opportunities for growth, practicing self-compassion, and adjusting expectations are coping strategies that can help manage setbacks and relapses. By using these strategies, individuals can stay motivated and make progress towards their healing goals.

Conclusion

The power of healing with time

Healing with time is a powerful process that allows individuals to recover from emotional, mental, and physical injuries. It is important to understand that healing is a journey, and it takes time to heal completely. Here are some ways that demonstrate the power of healing with time:

1. Healing with time provides a natural and holistic approach: Healing with time provides a natural and holistic approach to healing that allows individuals to process emotions, experiences, and physical injuries at their own pace.

2. It allows for emotional and mental processing: Healing with time allows for emotional and mental processing, which can help individuals gain insight, develop coping strategies, and move forward.

3. It promotes resilience: The process of healing with time can promote resilience by helping individuals develop skills to cope with future challenges.

4. It can lead to personal growth and development: The journey of healing with time can lead to personal growth and development by providing individuals with opportunities to learn, gain insight, and develop new perspectives.

5. It can improve overall well-being:

Healing with time can improve overall well-being by reducing stress, anxiety, and depression, improving physical health, and increasing feelings of happiness and contentment.

6. It can lead to a sense of empowerment: The process of healing with time can lead to a sense of empowerment by allowing individuals to take control of their healing journey, gain a sense of agency, and become more self-aware.

Healing with time is a powerful process that can provide natural and holistic approaches to emotional, mental, and physical healing. It allows individuals to process emotions and experiences, promotes resilience, leads to personal growth and development, improves overall well-being, and can lead to a sense of empowerment. It is important to remember that healing is a journey and takes time, but the benefits of healing with time are well worth the effort.

Encouragement to trust the process and prioritize self-care

Encouragement to trust the process and prioritize self-care is essential for individuals who are healing from emotional, mental, and physical injuries. It can be challenging to trust the process and prioritize self-care, especially when setbacks occur. However, here are some ways to encourage individuals to trust the process and prioritize self-care:

1. Celebrate progress: Celebrating progress, no matter how small,

can help individuals recognize the steps they have taken on their healing journey and encourage them to continue.

2. Practice self-compassion: Practicing self-compassion is essential for individuals who are healing. Being kind to oneself, acknowledging challenges and setbacks, and offering support can help individuals maintain a positive outlook.

3. Focus on the present: Focusing on the present moment can help individuals stay grounded and reduce anxiety about the future.

4. Seek support: Seeking support from family, friends, or professionals can provide individuals with a network of

people who understand their experiences and can offer guidance and encouragement.

5. Prioritize self-care: Prioritizing self-care is crucial for individuals who are healing. Engaging in activities that promote physical, emotional, and mental well-being can help individuals maintain balance and reduce stress.

6. Embrace patience: Embracing patience can be challenging, but it is necessary for individuals who are healing. Remembering that healing takes time and allowing oneself to trust the process can be powerful.

Encouraging individuals to trust the process and prioritize self-care is essential for those who are healing.

Celebrating progress, practicing self-compassion, focusing on the present, seeking support, prioritizing self-care, and embracing patience are all ways to support individuals on their healing journey. It is important to remember that healing takes time, and being kind and patient with oneself is key to achieving long-term healing and growth.